DASH DIET

The complete guide for the weight loss program, it reduces hypertension and blood pressure, low-calorie meals, healthy and tasty recipes for an easy prepare, you choose to improve your health and prevent diabetes

Adele Cummins

Legal & Disclaimer

You agree to accept all risks of using the information presented inside this book.

You agree that by continuing to read this book, where appropriate and/or necessary, you shall consult a professional (including but not limited to your doctor, attorney, or financial advisor or such other advisor as needed) before using any of the suggested remedies, techniques, or information in this book.

Table of Contents

Introduction

The needs of the accelerated pace of urban life, a greater awareness of health and the need to respect the environment, and a consideration of food as a source of experiences, pleasure, and entertainment all affect the food products we consume and the food trends we follow. The fast-paced life and the need to stay healthy and fit have given rise to a number of food trends in the 21st century. These diets can be divided into nine categories that, from the looks of it, will be extended and consolidated in the coming years. These trends are:

- Ephemeral Food

Among many urbanites, food consumption is conditioned by a hectic pace of life, with work and personal hours that leave no room for regular meals or time to sit in a restaurant. Hence, more and more people need food that is available at any time, as well as a place where they can meet their food needs instantly without losing out in terms of quality or nutrition.

- Food Awareness

An increasing number of people are committed to environmentally sustainable products and services that do not involve social or animal abuse in any link of the production chain.

- Personalized Health

The greater availability of knowledge on topics related to health and nutrition has led many people to personalize their diets according to their state of their health and the needs of each vital organ. These people are consumers who look for healthy products adapted to their specific needs.

This might mean consuming foods without salt or gluten, or foods with certain vitamins or protein contributions.

A Measure of One's Identity

Consumption has become a way to express one's personal identity, to define oneself or show oneself in public. This applies to clothes, mobile phones, or food. There is an audience that seeks food products or services to reinforce its identity.

- Simple and Intelligent

This trend has been around for a while. The frantic pace of life causes consumers to look for flexible, accessible solutions that save them time when cooking and that make their lives easier.

- Origin Does Matter

While some people seek the quickest or simplest foods and take advantage of globalization in terms of variety and diversity, another group of consumers prefers local goods and chooses to eat only what they are clear about, be it for environmental or social reasons.

- Food Experience

For a growing number of consumers, eating is much more than simply feeding the body. They look for food that provides them with a unique and memorable experience. The tendency to link everything that surrounds the world of food with emotional states, with fun, or with a search for new things is on the rise.

- **Participation**

New technologies favor a participative culture around food. Consumers are not satisfied to be merely recipients of food; they want to express their opinions, learn and influence the tastes and the creation of new products, and even affect the conditions of purchase. A very clear example is collaborative consumption platforms online.

- **Awareness**

The latest trend has led some consumers to bet on products, companies, and brands that promote or share their personal values, which are transparent, honest, or fun.

These nine trends are not mutually exclusive; some consumers respond to more than one or bet on one or the other depending on the moment. However, all kinds of food trends today fall into at least one of these subcategories.

Chapter 1-What is the Dash Diet?

Chances are that if you stay up to date on current health trends, you have already heard of the DASH Diet. DASH was first developed as a clearly defined, medically endorsed eating plan to reduce blood pressure in patients that were either hypertensive or at risk. As more and more people became aware of the eating plan, it became better known, not only for its disease fighting properties, but also because it is simply one of the most nutritionally sound programs around today. The foundation of the DASH Diet that is low in sodium, unhealthy fats, and cholesterol, while encouraging the increased consumption of high fiber foods that are rich in calcium, magnesium, and potassium. The result is an almost magical combination of foods that promotes optimal health.

Because the focus of the DASH Diet is primarily fresh vegetables, fruits, low fat dairy products and lean healthy proteins, it naturally lends itself to promoting healthy, lifelong weight loss. Because we are all individuals with varying health needs, the DASH Diet has evolved to include a couple of different versions. In this 14-day plan, we include what is known as Phase One and Phase Two. Phase one is a metabolism boosting and weight shedding jump start to the plan, for those who have weight loss as a primary health goal. Along with losing weight and becoming more heart healthy, following the DASH Diet will provide you increased energy, clearer mental focus, fewer side effects from chronic conditions and the natural glow of healthiness.

Once you read a little further in this book, you will discover (if you do not know already) that the DASH Diet is in no way a questionable dietary trend with just as many ill effects as positive ones. The DASH Diet has been approved and endorsed by The American Heart Association, The National Heart, Lung and Blood Institute, and the

Mayo Clinic, and it follows the American Governmental Dietary Guidelines. All of this on top of the fact that US News and World Report awarded the DASH Diet with the honor of being the top dietary plan for five years in a row. This is an amazing, effective diet and lifestyle that you can confidently present to your physician and the support people in your life. The only real question now is how you can integrate the DASH Diet into your life, and the answer is very simple.

The DASH Diet is built around common sense and well known healthy dietary principles, with an emphasis on food that is meant to appeal to a wide variety of ages, culinary lifestyles, and appetites. The ingredients you will use are simple, fresh, and no-fuss. There are only a few "rules" to keep in mind and it is a plan that is easily adapted to suit food allergies, sensitivities, and lifestyle choices, such as vegetarianism. This is the most well thought out, easy to follow, and intuitive plan that you will find today, and the benefits are many. Soon you will be on your way to becoming healthier and more energetic than you ever thought possible.

DASH Diet Guidelines

You know that the DASH Diet is a nutritional plan that is strongly focused on the consumption of fresh produce and lean, quality protein sources, and follows the United States Food Pyramid guidelines. Any dietary plan that focuses on these foods is bound to be a success, so what is it about the DASH Diet that makes it so effective, and one of the top diets recommended by physicians? The DASH diet looks not only at how generally healthy a food is, it goes further to look at the nutritional content—specifically nutrients such as calcium, potassium, and magnesium. This ensures that each day you get a combination of nutritional elements that promote the best possible state of well-being within your body. Following is a quick guideline of what to eat while following the DASH eating plan. These guidelines are based on an 1800-2000 calorie-a-day diet. The amount of calories you consume will depend upon your current body type, activity level and whether you currently have any weight loss goals, or whether an overall improvement in health is your primary concern. Determining your unique level of optimal calories considers many different factors. For this reason, it is best to discuss this with a physician or other qualified professional that can take your individual circumstances into account. Adjust these recommended servings appropriately based on your preferred daily calorie consumption. Also, keep in mind that during Phase One of the DASH Diet, grain and fruit consumption is limited and the suggested guidelines for those food groups apply to Phase Two of the plan.

Chapter 2- Why it is the best and true American diet

A diet based on unprocessed plants does not include meat, dairy or eggs. However, it is not the identical as a vegan diet, which is defined only by what it eliminates. A diet based on unprocessed plants is also defined by what it emphasizes: a large variety of unprocessed foods.

The term "unprocessed" in raw plant-based food describes foods that are minimally processed. This includes as many whole grain bowls of cereal, fruits, vegetables and legumes as you wish.

You do not need a calculator to count calories or carbohydrates. There is no need to avoid cooked foods. Convenience is not your enemy. You are allowed to consume frozen fruits and vegetables, as well as their canned counterparts (just be sure to find low sodium options). Insipidity is not a prerequisite. Go ahead and experiment with as many spices as you want. And finally, contrary to popular belief, a diet based on raw plants will not affect your budget. Many of your trusted staple foods (think of beans and potatoes) are among the most affordable foods in the market store. This diet does not require special items hidden in the healthy food section. It does not require agave pails or trolleys of cashews.

Many eventually renounce the label of "food or diet" in favor of "lifestyle". Maybe it's because our popular notion of diet has become very distorted and confusing. It involves a struggle; it poses each meal as a challenge to be overcome. A lifestyle with a diet based on raw plants is different. It is not a short-term punishment, charged with guilt. It is simply a return to unprocessed foods, rich flavors and natural health.

1. A plant-based diet also helps prevent certain types of cancer, reduces the incidence of heart disease and diabetes, cholesterolemia, hypertension, Alzheimer's, Parkinson's disease, rheumatoid arthritis, ulcers and vaginal infections. Are we still going?

A plant-centered diet has a positive effect on the prevention of abdominal fat accumulation, the appearance of acne, ageing, allergies, asthma, body odour, cellulite, eczema, metabolic syndrome and body weight control, just increasing the consumption of fruits and vegetables increases the chances of extending our life expectancy, but a life with higher quality in health. On the contrary, the consumption of meat and other foods of animal origin, such as dairy products, have shown that, due to its high content of saturated fats, arachidonic acid and Heme iron, life is shortened.

The consumption of meat, fish, dairy and eggs also increases the exposure to antibiotics, mercury and other heavy metals and xenoestrogens in fish and carcinogenic substances in meat that is formed when cooked at high temperatures.

Contrary to popular belief, most vegans get enough protein in their diet, consume more nutrients than the average omnivore, and usually maintain an adequate weight. There are only two vitamins that we cannot find in plant foods, these are vitamin D, which we obtain from exposure to the sun, and vitamin B12, produced by mycobacteria that live in the earth, and from which one must be supplemented.

2. Maintain Your Proper Weight

The evil of many is the accumulation of weight that one adds up over the years. As my colleague, Dr Mauricio González says, from the age of 22, the only thing that can grow is the belly or a tumour. So to prevent the birth of both follows a vegetable diet will be our ally.

The reality is that if we consume many vegetables in our dishes, the caloric contribution of these will decrease since on average, a cup of vegetables gives us between 10-50 kcal. And if above, we are replacing another fatty, sweet and processed foods with these ingredients, without a doubt you will be reducing the calories consumed at the end of the day, and you will even feel fuller since you will consume more fiber.

3. Eat Healthy and Economical

 Many people believe that eating healthy or foods of vegetable origin are expensive and resort to processed food or junk, "fast food" because they think it is the cheapest. Certainly, this is not reality.

Visiting a fast food restaurant such as Burger King and or Mc Donalds, to buy hamburgers, chips and sodas, will not be cheaper than buying 1 packet of lentils , 1 packet of rice, 1 onion and a bag of frozen spinach with what you can prepare a delicious and complete cooked for the whole family.

Also, as the saying goes, prevention is more suitable than cure, and in the United States, going to the doctor is for the privileged. In countries where to remove the appendix charge you $10,000, it is better to invest in buying organic and quality food, to go through surgery, pay the hospital bill, the rehabilitation therapist, be low and sooner or later start to Invest in preventive medicine (healthy food) to avoid another scare in your health.

The only thing you save by eating at these junk food restaurants is time, the time to cook. But believe me, once you're in the kitchen, you can prepare double the rations, freeze them, and have them for other days of the week. It's just about being practical and sometimes a little creative, playing with different spices, seasonal vegetables, and varying the cereal or legume.

Lentils, beans and peas are some of the cheapest foods with high nutritional value that you can find in the supermarket. When we talk about fruits and vegetables, we must always go for the options that are in season, and even buy extra when they are on offer and freeze them for when it is not their time. So you can do with blueberries and other berries, to have a good reserve of local production in winter.

4. Sustainability And Health Of The Planet

You need 15 kilos of cereals to obtain 1 kilo of beef, and 5 kilos to obtain 1 kilo of chicken meat. The majority of the grains that are cultivated worldwide are destined to the raising of the cattle, so we would be talking about a massive reduction of the consumption of water and energy if these cereals were for human consumption.

Did you know that half the water used in the United States is for livestock? 1,750 liters of water are needed to produce a 120g beef burger. In the case of milk, we are not talking about more beautiful numbers ... 3,800 liters of water are needed to produce 4 liters of cow's milk. An unsustainable system!

An article published in 2009 in Scientific American announced that the amount of beef consumed by an average American citizen at the end of the year produced the same amount of gas emissions as driving a car over 2,900km.

We usually blame the emission of cars, planes and factory fumes for being responsible for the greenhouse effect, but we never talk about the great weight that livestock has on this fact. About the FAO (Food and Agriculture Organization), livestock is responsible for 18% of the emissions of these gases, which is more than the sum of emissions by all means of transport combined.

The statistics say that if all Americans stopped eating a portion of chicken a week, we would save the same amount of CO2 emissions as if we were to eliminate 500,000 cars from the road. In fact, following a plant-based diet can reduce each's carbon footprint by up to 50%.

According to the International Livestock Research Institute, livestock activity occupies 46% of the land that exists on the planet. This activity is guilty of the deforestation of 91% of the Amazon rainforest, one of the main lungs of our planet, an oxygen emitter that helps us clean our atmosphere.

Another fact to which it's suggested that you pay attention and do the calculation yourself ..., 6,000 square meters of land can produce 170 kilos of meat or 16,800 kilos of plant foods.

5. Animal Cruelty

We all look away or change channels when we see images of slaughterhouses or tortured animals, it is important to be aware of reality.

As the pig grows, space is becoming tighter; they begin to develop sores on their skin from scratches with the walls of the cage. They urinate and defecate through the grooves of the cage, creating an atmosphere full of ammonia, a precursor of lung diseases. Once the sow gives birth, it is separated from its young and returns to its cage until it is time to go to the slaughterhouse.

These are some of the praxis that is used to save money and increase meat production, but at what cost? Pigs are even smarter animals than the dogs we have at home, with the only difference that we have never considered having a pig as a pet.

6. Hunger In The World

The world produces sufficient food to feed 10 billion people. The United States alone could feed 800 million people with cereals that are grown to feed livestock. Hunger is not a problem of scarcity; it is a problem of allocation and distribution.

Chapter 3- Organizing and initializing the daily meal plan

An average adult consumes about 6 grams of sodium a day. This could be in the form of table salt or preserved foods that are rich in sodium. However, even if this seems to be the usual amount of sodium that people take in every day, it does not seem to be the recommended one. An average adult needs only 2 grams of salt per day that is equivalent to about 1 tablespoon of table salt. From this fact alone, you may have already known that you are exceeding your daily total sodium needs.

Sodium is one of the major electrolytes in the body that play very important roles in maintaining body homeostasis. It is the major extracellular cation (a positively-charged particle) of the body. To better understand this definition of sodium, here is a brief explanation of how the circulatory system works.

The circulatory system is composed of the heart, which is the body's main pump, and its blood vessels, which are networks of pipes and tubings that serve as the passageways of blood. The heart pumps out blood into the general circulation, while the blood vessels deliver them to the cells. In order to pump out blood into the system, the heart must be able to overcome the pressure inside the major arteries, most specifically the aorta. If the pressure in the aorta is increased, then the heart must work harder to be able to overcome the pressure. The aorta then receives the blood and delivers it to the organs and tissues through a complex network of vessels. The general rule is, the further away the artery is from the heart, the lower the pressure gets. However, one needs to maintain the pressure at a certain point because this helps the blood to be propelled back to the heart. The maintenance of the pressure becomes the function of the muscles, especially in the lower extremities, and the fluid forces, as explained by Starling's Law. The muscles serve as pumps to push the blood back to the heart through contractions. When you are immobile, there is a lesser amount of blood that goes back to your heart.

There are two forces that keep the pressure inside the blood vessels in equilibrium: the hydrostatic pressure and the oncotic pressure. The hydrostatic pressure is the force generated by the pumping of the heart, which pushes the water out into the interstitial space, while the oncotic pressure is the force generated by the electrolytes and proteins present in the blood, such as sodium and albumin, respectively, that pulls the water in the interstitial space back into the blood vessels. When the levels of sodium and albumin increase, as a result of an increase in intake or a decrease in excretion, more water is being pulled back into the circulation.

The blood vessels, with the plasma inside, comprise a part of the extracellular compartment of the body. The other extracellular compartment is the interstitial space, or the space in between cells. This is the compartment where sodium is mostly found, which is one of the regulators of fluid in the compartment. On the other hand, the compartment inside the cells is called the intracellular space. As mentioned previously, when the sodium levels in the extracellular compartment rises, there is a corresponding increase in the fluid level in the same compartment. How does this happen? This is because the sodium exerts a pulling effect on the fluids, specifically those located in the intracellular space. The fluids then shift from the intracellular into the intravascular space, increasing the blood volume present in the vessels. As the blood volume increases, the cardiac output proportionately increases. And as mentioned in the previous chapter, cardiac output is a factor in the maintenance of blood pressure. BP increases proportionately with CO. The rule of thumb is, wherever the sodium, the water follows.

What happens to the cell that loses fluid? Typically, the cells shrink with loss of fluid. But when the loss is too great, the cells die. This then causes an alteration in the body's processes, which may later on present as a disease. Not only that, sodium, as mentioned before, can cause stiffening of the vessels that may cause an increase in the TPR, thus, an increase in BP.

Because of the effects of sodium on the blood volume and on the blood vessel walls, sodium must be adequately regulated. In response to this, the body makes use of various mechanisms to 1) regulate the amount of sodium in the body; 2) to regulate its excretion; and 3) to regulate your sodium intake.

When you take in salty foods, you normally feel thirsty. This is because of the shrinkage of cells that is caused by the shift of fluids from the intracellular into the extracellular space. The hypothalamus then senses this shift and sends a signal to your brain that you need to drink in order to counteract these effects. Increasing your fluid intake replenishes the fluid stores of your intracellular compartment and you no longer feel the thirst.

This goes hand in hand with the regulation of its excretion. The major organ responsible for excreting sodium is the kidney, which filters the sodium out from the blood and sends it out when you urinate. An increase in the sodium levels in the blood causes a corresponding increase in its filtration and excretion.

The body can also regulate the amount of sodium in the body by exchanging it with other electrolytes. This is accomplished through pump exchangers that exchange one electrolyte for another electrolyte to enter the cell. An example of this is the sodium-hydrogen exchanger. When levels of sodium go up, this exchanger present on the surface of the cells takes up sodium and releases hydrogen, which is another cation. The same is true for the sodium-calcium exchanger. When sodium goes up, the exchanger takes up sodium and releases calcium. This way, the serum sodium levels return to normal.

If there are mechanisms to reduce or to regulate sodium levels, why do people still get hypertension? This is because these mechanisms are only efficient up to a certain point. It has been explained earlier that the excretion of sodium is the function of the kidneys. True, BUT with excessive rise in sodium levels, this mechanism becomes altered. Here's how.

High blood levels of sodium trigger vasoconstriction, and one of the consequences of this event is a decrease in blood flow to the organs. One of the major organs whose function is very dependent on the amount of blood that it receives is the kidney. A decrease in renal blood flow causes a chain of events that ultimately leads to sodium retention. When the kidneys sense that it is not getting an adequate amount of blood flow, one of its cells, called the juxtaglomerular cells, would produce renin, an enzyme that would activate angiotensinogen to angiotensin I. Up to this point, there are no major changes in the body. The major change occurs when angiotensin I is converted to angiotensin II in the lungs by another enzyme, called angiotensin-converting enzyme (ACE). This substance is one of the potent vasoconstrictors known, thus causing more vasoconstriction. Angiotensin II causes the release of aldosterone, a hormone that functions to conserve sodium. As a result, sodium is not excreted and fluids are retained. This leads to a vicious cycle that further compromises sodium regulation and blood pressure.

Because of the various effects of sodium, the DASH diet recommends that you keep your sodium intake at a minimum. If you want to cut your sodium intake, it is necessary that you know which foods contain a lot of sodium and which ones contain less.

Generally, preserved, canned and processed foods are rich in sodium. One slice of bacon, for instance, contains approximately 150 mg of sodium, while a slice of ham has even more sodium with 1300 mg! A slice of bacon and ham already contain the amount of sodium that you need for one day! Other foods rich in sodium are white bread, pancakes, canned tuna and dairy products like butter and cheese. If you are a carnivorous type of person and you don't want to give up meat, try chicken. The part of the chicken with the lowest amount of sodium is the chicken breast, with only 80 mg of sodium per slice. A roasted pork loin also has less sodium, with only 65 mg per slice. Other foods that are low in sodium are vegetables and fruits. A slice of cucumber only has 2 mg, a cup of eggplant has 5 mg and a cup of beans has 5 mg. Medium sized apples, bananas and oranges all have 1 mg each, while each cup of grapes and strawberries has 2 mg!

When you are making a meal plan, you can consider these sodium levels. You can opt to increase your vegetable and fruit servings with a moderate amount of chicken and pork and lower your servings of cured pork. Table salt, soy sauce, broths and monosodium glutamate are undeniably some of the best sources of sodium, so cut down on these, too. You can replace them with herbs instead. If you want to eat vegetables that are moderately high in sodium, like spinach, broccoli and beets, you can boil them first and discard the broth before adding them to your dish.

Here is a simple recipe to start off your day with a low-sodium meal:

Nutty Banana Oatmeal

Ingredients:

1 medium sized banana, peeled and sliced

½ cup rolled oats

½ cup water

1 cup almonds, chopped

Procedure:

1. Heat the pan over low heat and cook rolled oats with water for 3 minutes.

2. Remove from heat and transfer to a bowl.

3. Add sliced bananas and chopped almonds.

4. Mix well.

Note: You need not add salt and sugar to this recipe.

Work on Your Minerals
DASH diet recommends an adequate intake of calcium, magnesium and potassium. These minerals are some of the major electrolytes in the body and they function to regulate different body processes.

A. Calcium

Though calcium is famous for its functions on the bones and teeth, recent studies show that calcium is also needed for the proper functioning of the heart. 99% of the calcium in the body is located in the bones and teeth, and the remaining 1% stays in the blood stream. This 1% functions primarily for nerve transmission and muscular contractions.

The heart is composed of cardiac muscles that function to pump blood out into the circulation. When the cardiac muscles get weak, there is less blood that is delivered to the different parts of the body, and thus may trigger reactions from the different organs that may cause a rapid rise in blood pressure. Vasoconstriction occurs, release of renin by the kidneys occurs and the heart may undergo dysrhythmic episodes, all of which may elevate blood pressure.

Calcium is one of the minerals being attributed to the proper contraction of the heart. Normally, each skeletal muscle fiber contains calcium stores that are released in the presence of appropriate stimuli. Once released, calcium will cause a strong contraction of the muscle fibers. The calcium has a different effect on the cardiac muscle cells. In the presence of calcium, the heart undergoes refractory period for every beat that it does. Do you ever wonder why the heart beats in a certain coordinated fashion? When you listen to your heartbeat, you will hear the "lub" and "dub" one after the other in a regular rhythm. This is because of the presence of calcium. For example, the heart beats to pump the blood into the aorta. The calcium will then try to control the heart muscles and let the heart relax for a certain period of time, usually not lasting more than a few seconds. Even with the presence of another stimulus, the heart remains in a refracted state.

This refractory mechanism of calcium has a lot of benefits for the heart. First, it lets the heart rest for a while, thus preventing muscular fatigue. It also gives the heart ample time to replenish its energy and to fill its chambers with blood. This period is called diastole and it is also during this period that the heart gets its blood supply from the coronary arteries. Imagine if the heart beats continuously without refraction. There is less blood pumped out and less blood being delivered to the muscles of the heart. When this happens, the body will initiate compensatory mechanisms that may lead to blood pressure elevation.

An average adult needs to take in 1 gram of dietary calcium every day. Foods rich in calcium include milk, yogurt, sardines, anchovies, soy beans and spinach. To get adequate amounts of calcium, it is also necessary to take in foods rich in vitamin D. This fat-soluble vitamin enhances the absorption of calcium in the intestines. The recommended daily allowance for vitamin D for an average adult is 600 to 800 IU. Foods rich in vitamin D are eggs, salmon, sesame seeds, liver and fortified foods. Milk and sardines are also good sources.

Calcium absorption decreases with age, with only about 2% of the dietary calcium being absorbed in late adulthood. This stresses the importance of eating vitamin D- and calcium-rich foods to counteract the age- induced decrease in absorption. A glass of milk and a cup of yogurt both contain approximately 300 mg of calcium, while a can of sardines contains approximately 250 mg.

Here is a simple recipe to guide you with your calcium intake:

Salmon Fillet

Ingredients:

½ kilo salmon fillet, sliced into strips

1 cup low-fat milk

1 cup fortified flour

Olive oil, for frying

2 eggs, scrambled

Dash of pepper

1 tbsp. Rosemary leaves, chopped

Procedure:

1. Prepare the fillet: Add rosemary leaves and dash of pepper to scrambled eggs and soak the salmon strips for 1 minute.

2. Roll the strips over the flour until well-coated.

3. Heat the pan and oil over medium heat.

4. Fry the fillet until golden brown.

5. Drain the oil from the fish before serving.

B. Potassium

Potassium, in contrast to sodium, is the major intracellular cation, and just like calcium, it has beneficial effects to the heart. It functions for nerve transmission, maintenance of fluid homeostasis and in lowering blood pressure.

Potassium is an electrolyte that has an antagonistic effect to sodium. Whenever potassium is high, sodium is low, and vice versa. How does potassium lower the blood pressure? First, potassium keeps the fluid inside the cells. Recall that fluid overload can cause an increase in cardiac output and a corresponding increase in blood pressure. With the potassium inside the cells, it indirectly keeps the fluid and the blood volume in the extracellular space at a constantly normal level.

Potassium is also needed by the heart for its contraction. When the heart contracts, it undergoes a series of depolarizations and repolarizations. Depolarization refers to the contraction, while repolarization is the relaxation of the muscle. These events are the function of an active pump called sodium- potassium (Na-K) pump. When the heart receives the stimulus from its pacemaker to contract, sodium goes into the cell and potassium passively diffuses out. This part constitutes the depolarization of the heart. However, the balance needs to be restored such that potassium is kept inside the cell, while the sodium is kept at the extracellular space. This is accomplished by the pump that pumps sodium out and allows the potassium to move into the cell, thus restoring it to normal. As potassium moves into the cell, the heart undergoes repolarization.

Taking this concept into context, without potassium, the heart remains in a contracted state. How does this happen? When the sodium goes inside the cell, a proportionate number of potassium goes out. The potassium that goes out of the cell is expected to go back with the help of the Na-K pump. Without potassium to go out of and back to the cell, sodium remains inside the cell, prolonging its contraction. With little amount of potassium, the heart is only able to repolarize for a shorter period of time. This event can be dangerous to your heart because it can deplete your heart of its energy. With a hypocontracting heart, the body would again institute compensatory measures to increase cardiac output at the expense of your blood pressure.

Potassium also has some renal protective effects. It has been said that kidney plays a crucial role in water balance and in maintaining normal blood pressure. Potassium is reported to decrease blood pressure by maintaining good kidney function. Studies show that potassium can prevent formation of kidney stones by acidifying the urine. The acidity helps dissolve the stones, thus, eliminate the risk of altered kidney functions.

Foods rich in potassium include bananas, avocados, potatoes, sweet potatoes, kiwi, plum and tomatoes. An average adult needs to take in 5 grams of potassium a day. 1 cup of spinach contains 800 mg of potassium, 1 cup tomatoes have 450 mg, 1 potato can contain as much as 900 mg and 1 cup avocadoes contain approximately 700 mg.

Here is a simple recipe you can follow to boost your potassium intake!

Banana Avocado Salsa

Ingredients:

1 cup banana, sliced

1 cup avocado, sliced

4 tbsp. lemon juice

1 tbsp. chopped cilantro

Procedure:

1. Combine all the ingredients.

2. You may eat this with wheat bread.

C. Magnesium

Magnesium is one of the minerals that people used to ignore but recent studies link magnesium with lower blood pressure, less incidence of stroke and heart attack. Magnesium is an intracellular cation. And together with potassium, they create a balance between the two fluid compartments. Magnesium is also shown to play a major role in electrolyte balance as a decrease or a decrease in this mineral can significantly cause a shift in electrolyte levels. One example of this scenario is hypokalemia. Though hypokalemia or low blood levels of potassium, is attributed to poor intake, it is predominantly caused by an increase in its excretion. Surprisingly, excretion of potassium is modulated by magnesium. With less amounts of magnesium, more and more potassium gets to be excreted out of the body through the urine. Thus, in correcting hypokalemia, it is necessary that you also correct hypomagnesemia.

Magnesium can also lower blood pressure by regulating calcium activity. It keeps calcium in the cells so it can maintain its functions. Other substances being regulated by magnesium include vitamin D, which is also necessary for calcium homeostasis, vitamin K, which is essential for clotting mechanisms, zinc and copper. A decrease in the blood levels of magnesium can trigger a corresponding decrease in the blood levels of these substances, creating imbalances and alterations that may be life-threatening in severe cases.

One of the major functions of magnesium is in energy production. It acts as a coenzyme in many metabolic processes, thus helps in the generation of Adenosine triphosphate (ATP), called the cell's energy currency. A cell won't be able to function without this substance, and the heart is not an exemption. The heart, as you have previously learned, needs adequate amount of energy to perform its sole function, which is to pump blood. Once the muscles of the heart have been weakened, a series of events can occur that may be deleterious to one's life. Heart attack, heart failure, stroke and multiple organ failure are just some of the complications of an inadequate energy production in the heart muscles. Hence, lowered blood magnesium levels can predispose you to a lot of life- threatening conditions.

Magnesium is present in foods where calcium and vitamin D are also found. An average adult needs 350 to 450 mg of magnesium daily. Most common sources of magnesium are dark green leafy vegetables, like broccoli and spinach, which contain approximately 150 to 160 grams of magnesium; a half cup of seeds and nuts, like sunflower and squash seeds, contains about 600 mg; a cup of beans contains about 150 mg; and a cup of dark chocolate contains about 450 mg.

If you want to jumpstart your magnesium habit today, try this simple recipe:

Chicken Potato Croquette

Ingredients:

1 kilo potato, peeled and boiled

1 cup non-fat milk

½ cup grated low-fat cheese

2 cups chicken fillet, in thin strips

3 eggs, scrambled

2 cups bread crumbs

½ cup celery

Canola oil

Procedure:

1. Mash the boiled potatoes

2. Add non-fat milk and celery. Mix well.

3. Flatten mashed potatoes onto your palm and top with strips of chicken and cheese.

4. Roll the mashed potato with the chicken and the cheese in the center.

5. Dip the rolled potato in to the scrambled eggs.

6. Roll over bread crumbs until well- coated.

7. Deep fry until golden brown.

Chapter 4- Types of simple physical exercises to follow with the diet

The DASH diet works more effectively in lowering blood pressure when you exercise more. Given the incredible benefits of exercise for your health, this is not surprising.

A bit of exercise, for example, can relieve stress and burn the necessary calories. You can lower your blood pressure in part by regularly exercising.

Rest assured, you don't have to go to the gym. Moderately concentrated forms of movement do you very well.

Examples of moderately intensive movement are:

- Nice walk, for example, during lunch.
- Running, half an hour in the evening. Then take a nice shower, and you will feel reborn!
- Cycling, from and to work. Super easy.
- Swimming.
- Household chores. Never thought that vacuuming your house and the windows would be good to keep your blood pressure in order?

DASHes

The DASH diet can, therefore, be an easy and effective way to lower your blood pressure. The diet can also cause you to lose weight. But this is not the intention. You do eat healthier if, for example, you eat a lot of processed food and regularly open a bag of crisps and come to a fast food restaurant.

The fresh vegetables, fruit and nuts do a lot of good. What would be disagreeing is so much with the DASH diet is limiting dietary fats and protein sources such as beef. This makes the DASH diet look like an impoverished diet. And you would not advise that yourself.

Over the past 40 years, a particular researcher started eating fewer fats. Take a look at what this has yielded! Being overweight is a true epidemic. And that's not all, being overweight increases the risk of heart disease, diabetes 2, osteoporosis and more lifestyle diseases.

Eating fewer fats is, therefore, not a solution.

You will soon know how to:

- Lose weight (without feeling hungry and calorie-counting). Pounds!
- Healthy and tasty food
- Get fit and energetic again

High Blood Pressure? The Dash Diet Has Proven To Be Efficient

The number of people with high blood pressure is increasing worldwide. Research shows again that the so-called DASH diet has proven to be effective and lowers blood pressure.

The DASH diet was devised by the American professor Lawrence Appel and stood for Dietary Approaches to Stop Hypertension. The core of the diet is a diet with lots of fruit, vegetables and low-fat dairy — also, mainly whole-grain products, chicken, fish and nuts. Red meat, confectionery and sugary soft drinks are kept to a minimum. The diet is extremely popular in the United States and has been voted the best diet several times (US News). The diet closely follows the guidelines of the Health Council and the Nutrition Center.

New investigation

The research shows once again that people with a slightly higher and too high blood pressure benefit greatly from the DASH diet and a diet low in salt. American researchers compared three dietary patterns with each other for 4 weeks:

1. A diet with high versus low salt

2. The DASH diet versus a control diet and

3. A combination: low salt + DASH diet versus a high salt/control diet.

The most effect was achieved in people with high blood pressure with a (combined) DASH diet low in salt, with lots of vegetables, fruit and low-fat dairy. The effect turned out to be just as great as the effect that can be achieved with blood pressure-lowering drugs. People with somewhat lower blood pressure also benefit from the diet.

Risk

Factor High blood pressure is an important risk factor for cardiovascular disease. This risk increases as blood pressure increases. Eating less salt can help to lower blood pressure. We only need 1 to 3 grams of salt per day. However, on average, we get 9 grams of salt. 80% of this is processed in industrially processed food such as bread, cheese and meat products. 20% is appended by the consumer himself.

If everyone in the Netherlands were to eat 3 grams less salt per day, 1,500 deaths and 6,000 new cases of cardiovascular disease could be prevented each year.

Study design

More than 400 American participants with an average age of 48 and a (slightly) elevated blood pressure participated in the study. They did not use medication. What is new is that the effects on the systolic blood pressure of the participants were analyzed at the start of the food experiments.

By eating less salt, systolic blood pressure decreased by 3.2 mmHg in the low blood pressure group (120-130 mmHg) and 7.0 mmHg in the high blood pressure group (150-160 mmHg). The DASH diet reduced blood pressure by 4.5 mmHg and 10.6 mmHg in both groups, respectively. The combination diet had the greatest effect, which increased with increasing blood pressure: a decrease of 5.3 mmHg in the group of people with low blood pressure (120-130 mmHg), a decrease of 7.5 mmHg in those with blood pressure of 130-139 mmHg, a decrease of 9.7 mmHg for those with blood pressure between 140-149 mmHg and a decrease of 20.8 mmHg for those with blood pressure 150-160 mmHg.

Chapter 5-How to best initiate the second phase of meals

There are two phases to the DASH Diet, Phase One and Phase Two. Phase One is the jump start phase that is intended to reset your metabolism. This phase is high in protein and is restrictive in terms of sugars and starches. Traditionally, this phase of the plan is meant to last the first two weeks, giving your body ample time to adjust to the new style of eating. Considering that this is an all-inclusive 14-day plan, we have shortened that phase to last the first seven days, and then introduce you to Phase Two of the plan which includes fresh fruits, legumes, and grains. You will find that during the Phase One period you will consume more than the initially recommended amounts of lean meats, low fat dairy and nuts. This is to make sure you are provided with ample caloric intake and variety during this phase. If you choose, you may extend this to a 21-day plan and stretch out Phase One into two weeks simply by repeating it. Alternatively, if you do not wish to participate in Phase One and would prefer to start out on Phase Two for health benefits that do not include rapid initial weight loss, this is perfectly acceptable also. Simple go straight ahead to Phase Two and repeat for two weeks in a row.

This plan is based on an 1800-2000 calorie-per-day menu, and is meant to include foods that will provide you with all of the essential nutrients. If weight loss is your primary goal, you may wish to cut the calories somewhat under the advice of a medical professional. Keep in mind that the high protein, low carbohydrate nature of Phase One means that you can consume more calories and still lose weight. The point is to increase your metabolism, not discourage it by restricting your calories too severely.

A couple of things to keep in mind during the 14-day plan: First of all, substitutions are acceptable. This isn't a rigid plan where you must eat certain foods without deviating from the plan. This is a lifestyle change, and it needs to fit in your life. That isn't going to happen if you are attempting to eat foods that you don't like or skipping meals and snacks to avoid them. The DASH Diet emphasizes foods that are rich in calcium, magnesium, and potassium. If you are going to substitute, the only rule is that the food you are substituting with is similar in nutritional content, especially in regard to those three nutrients. With that in mind, studies have shown that we gain the most from nutrients when we receive them from their original food sources, rather than taking them in supplement form. If you have a food intolerance or are unable to eat certain foods, then it is acceptable to supplement. Otherwise, strive to get all of your daily vitamin and minerals from your diet rather than a pill.

The DASH diet was formulated to address the factors that may lead to uneventful complications. Some of those factors have already been mentioned, like sodium and cholesterol. The other factors will be discussed in the next few chapters of the book. It is essential to take note that the DASH diet is not a one-time approach. It needs constancy, patience and commitment in order to achieve your goal. Getting started with it requires motivation and determination but it won't be as difficult if you know and follow these simple guidelines.

1. Take it slowly.
If this diet is a surprise to you, don't panic. You don't have to immediately adopt it. If applying it in a step-by-step process is what works for you, then go ahead. Because of the many factors that this diet encompasses, it is impossible for anyone to do them all at the same time. You can start with your sodium intake. If you love salty foods, it is high time to cut down your intake of these, BUT it is not necessary that you do it right away. If your daily salt intake amounts to ten tablespoons daily, which is a lot more than what is

recommended, you can start to lower it to nine tablespoons today. You can probably try this for a week, then lower it by one tablespoon every day for the next week.

The same is true when you don't love eating vegetables and you are a carnivorous type of person. You can start adding one vegetable at a time in your meals until such time that you get used to it.

2. Substitute.

In this day and age, different food products are already being sold in the market that can serve as substitutes for the unhealthy ones. If you love drinking milk in the morning or at night and you don't want to cut your intake, try the low-fat or non-fat milk products. Other dairy products like cheese and butter now have low-fat counterparts. Check them out. These products help lower your blood cholesterol. If you want a tasty dish without using salt, try herbs, like rosemary, basil, and thyme. They don't only make your meal savory, but healthy as well.

3. Eliminate.

Checking your kitchen, most especially your fridge, for healthy and unhealthy foods is the next best thing to do. Using the principles of hypertension and the DASH diet, which foods do you think should already be eliminated? Keep your vegetables, fruits and lean meat; eliminate sweets, high fat and salty foods. Doing this frees you from future temptations of eating the unhealthy ones. From here, you can already plan your meals with just the healthy foods in mind.

4. Make a meal plan.

To make adopting the DASH diet easier, it is better to have a meal plan ready and follow it. Plan meals for breakfast, lunch, dinner and snacks enough for the whole week so you are guided with the foods that you eat. This also helps you balance your diet out. Plan for a meal that is composed of grains, vegetables and fruits, fish and meat, and limit foods that are sweet and fatty.

5. Prepare a list.

When shopping for your ingredients, it is wise to have a list of what you are going to buy based on your meal plan. Be faithful to your list. This helps you avoid buying those which are unnecessary and unhealthy that can only blow up your expenses and take up too much space in your fridge.

Chapter 6-Be aware of what you are eating

Although some people like to talk about their diets, you may not want the whole world to know that you are on a diet. Studies show that telling others about your goals can make you less likely to achieve them. The sense of satisfaction you get from revealing your intention, like losing weight through a diet, can cause you to have a premature feeling of complacency.

Resort to distraction and avoidance

Change the subject, so you do not have to talk about food and diet when you talk to someone. If you discover yourself in a condition where diets emerge as a topic of conversation between friends and colleagues, use distracting tactics to change the subject, comment on the television show or the latest movies. Focus on the gossip of the office or the latest mutual friends' news. Changing the subject so as not to talk about food or diets will help you not to talk about your diet or your eating habits.

Take into account that it may be useful to share your diet with close friends or relatives, as they can serve as a form of support and encouragement. Instead of avoiding the issue when talking to people who are close to you, you may need to consider being open about your diet so you can feel that you are not alone or that you do not have to be ashamed.

Prepare an ambiguous excuse. Think of an ambiguous excuse in case someone asks you about your diet, especially if someone has done it recently and you have had to change the subject unnaturally. It can be something like "I'm just taking care of what I eat" or "I'm avoiding some food groups".

While thinking about an ambiguous excuse can be useful, you should try not to lie when someone asks you about your weight. For example, it would not be a good idea to say something like "The doctor has told me that I am allergic to carbohydrates" if it is not true that the doctor has made that diagnosis. Using a false excuse can indicate that you are ashamed of your eating habits and that you try to hide that you are dieting by lying to others. Also, it can be counterproductive and cause problems if someone sees you eating carbohydrates.

Look at the menu in advance if you are going to eat on the street. To avoid the waiter's awkward sway when you're in a restaurant, prepare to eat on the street by looking at the menu in advance on the store's website. In this way, you can read the entire menu and create a meal that meets your dietary needs without pressure, instead of doing it right there and in person.

If you eat at someone's house, you may have to ask the cook at home what she plans to cook. So, maybe you can suggest some dishes that can be adapted to your planned meal and that allow you to continue with your diet. While the cook may not accept to make a special meal for you, at least you will be prepared for the meal, and you will know what to eat when you sit down to eat.

Eating can only be a lonely and unhealthy experience, especially if you do it every day every time you eat. You may need to consider eating with people who do not question your diet or who do not ask personal questions about your eating habits as an alternative to not eating all meals alone. They can be friends who are also on a diet or people you've met through a weight loss program.

Focus on eating smart and healthy

Take a lot of water will not only keep you healthy and hydrated, but it can also act as an appetite suppressant. Drink plenty of water throughout the day to prevent your stomach from being empty, which can lead to high levels of hunger and the urge to eat. By drinking plenty of water, you can focus on staying hydrated and not on a diet.

You should also drink a glass of water before eating so that your stomach is fuller and you can eat smaller portions during the meal. This measure can help you eat more healthily.

Sandwiches such as raw almonds, dark chocolate and vegetable sticks with peanut butter or hummus can keep you full and give you energy between meals. You can also cut fruits such as apples, pears and bananas to have healthy snacks that do not cause a sugar collapse during the day.

Plan your meals. It has been found that eating distractedly and without planning leads to weight gain and unfruitful diets. Avoid it by planning your meals for the week. Go shopping at the beginning of the week (or the weekend if you work during the weekdays) so that you have all the necessary ingredients to prepare healthy meals at home that fit your diet.

You can organize meals according to a specific caloric intake per day or to a goal of weight loss. Try to plan your meals based on your daily caloric intake, which is based on age, weight and level of physical activity. Remember that each person will have a different caloric intake and that no diet can meet the dietary needs of all people.

Practice eating attentively. Another key component to practicing healthy eating habits is to be aware of how you eat, as well as what you eat. Numerous people tend to eat in front of the television or absentmindedly and do not pay attention to how much they eat. Instead of eating in front of the television, try to sit down and focus on the food as you eat, taking the time to save it. In this way, you can swallow and digest each bite and control the amount you eat.

To practice eating carefully, use a timer when you sit down to eat. Set the timer in 20 minutes and try to use all the time available to eat a meal.

You can decide to eat with your non-dominant hand, so you are forced to slow down when you eat and make an effort to lift and chew each bite. You can also reflect on what is needed to produce the food, such as a butcher to prepare meat or a farmer to grow vegetables and grains.

If you tend to drink a lot of coffee or enjoy a few drinks once in a while, try drinking a glass of water between each cup of coffee or each drink. In this way, you will stay hydrated and limit the pangs of hunger.

Visit a doctor if you think you have an eating disorder. Hiding the diet by resorting to exaggerated excuses, spitting food on napkins or not eating with other people are signs of an eating disorder such as bulimia or anorexia. These disorders are often due to the association of food with a high level of anxiety and anxiety. The following are some other symptoms of an eating disorder:

Do not eat anything at all

Cut food into small pieces or dilate eating time

Eat very fast or very slow, and then expel food by vomiting or using laxatives in excess

Eat without cutlery or cutlery that is not appropriate for food

Exercise intensely after each meal

Count calories and control eating habits obsessively

If you think you develop an eating disorder, you should talk to close friends and family. You should also consider seeking professional help from a doctor or a psychotherapist who specializes in eating disorders.

Determine if you want to share your success. If the diet is over and you have achieved your goals, determine if you want to share your success with friends and family. After all, people probably notice that you have lost weight and wish to celebrate with you.

Chapter 7-Tips, tricks and recipes to follow to avoid deviation

Some tips to follow this diet can be useful to organize the daily menus:

- Use various herbs and spices to replace table salt.
- Avoid smoked meats, sausages, canned, processed or preserved.
- Choose lean red meats, chicken without skin and little fat fish.
- Serve always moderate portions in the main meals and appetizers.
- Avoid frozen meals, soups and concentrated broths and salad dressings.
- Start the day with a good breakfast based on low-sodium cereals and without added salt.
- Cook the pasta, rice and other cereals without salt.
- Prefer water to replace soda with high sugar content.
- Limit the consumption of industrially processed foods that have a high salt content.

Example of the DASH Diet Menu

Here is an example of a DASH Diet menu that equals 1 day and contributes approximately 1800. To get better results, it is important to drink at least 8 glasses of water daily.

Example of DASH Diet Menu

Breakfast

1 cup of tea with skim milk and sweetener.

1 slice of toasted wheat bread

½ banana

Midmorning

1 natural yoghurt skimmed

½ cup of whole grains without sugar.

lunch

200 grs. Grilled skinless chicken with oregano.

1 salad of ½ cucumber, ½ tomato, ½ onion and lettuce leaves with 1 teaspoon of olive oil tea and without salt.

2 slices of wheat bread.

Mid-afternoon

1 cup of fruit salad without sugar.

1 cup of tea with skim milk and sweetener.

1 glass of orange juice

50 grs. of raisins of grapes.

50 grs. of almonds.

Dinner

200 grs. of grilled fish.

½ cup cooked brown rice without salt.

1 slice of wheat bread

1 piece of fruit

Variants of the DASH Diet

As the DASH Diet was created for the prevention and treatment of hypertension, there are numerous similar plans that not only have food as the main factor but also how to cook and preserve them.

In reality, there is no ideal food plan for hypertensive people, and that is why the DASH Diet is so well known that, in addition to being healthy, it provides enough nutrients that meet daily needs to stay fit and enjoys good health.

The role of diet is essential to prevent and treat high blood pressure being the cornerstone that supports the treatment of cardiovascular diseases.

Reduce the consumption of salt is the main measure for anyone who wants to prevent hypertension or for those who have already been diagnosed as hypertensive.

The daily salt needs for anyone so it is recommended to use less salt when cooking food and as much as possible replace it with pepper, herbs, garlic, lemon juice or spices.

Other recommendations for a diet for hypertensive patients other than DASH is to choose olive oil, products with little sodium in their industrial preparation, avoiding smoked or very salty meats, sausages in general and especially ham or bacon and when the restriction in the consumption of salt is greater can replace the common salt by potassium or magnesium.

An alternative diet to the DASH is the dietary treatment of the HTA that consists of

the reduction in the consumption of salt, greater ingestion of vegetables, fruits, legumes, fish, olive oil and foods that contain little fat.

The HTA diet also recommends limiting the consumption of alcohol and exciting substances such as caffeine that produce a significant increase in blood pressure. The allowed is less than 30 grams of alcohol per day for men and less than 20 grams for women and no more than two or three coffees a day.

This dietary HTA treatment recommends improving healthy lifestyle habits such as exercising, not smoking and controlling weight.

ADVANTAGES AND DISADVANTAGES OF THE DASH DIET

The DASH Diet has been designed especially for patients with hypertension but is also suitable for weight loss because it is recommended to eat fresh foods such as fruits and vegetables, low-fat dairy and restricted carbohydrates, limited consumption of salt and good daily hydration, definitely a healthy life at any stage of life.

Advantages of the DASH Diet control hypertension and help you lose weight

- Control and lower blood pressure and the bad cholesterol rate without resorting to medications.

- It is not necessary to count calories but to focus more on the food you eat every day to also lose weight.
- Accelerates metabolism, thanks to a change in eating habits.
- It avoids suffering the yo-yo effect or rebound common to many other diets.

Disadvantages of the DASH Diet to control blood pressure and lose weight

It is a diet high in fibre and can cause bloating.

It can cause constipation so you should drink enough water daily.

Recipes of the DASH Diet

The DASH Diet has been honored in 2012 and 2014 as the best diet to prevent and control high blood pressure according to a report published by US News & World Report.

There are numerous recipes for meals as well as snacks or snacks that are very useful when organizing the daily menu to carry out this diet. These are simple dishes, easy to prepare and with a lot of flavors and then we share some of them.

Chapter 8-How to maintain weight lost with these techniques

Losing weight is a typical aim for many people. Losing weight and being able to maintain a healthy level will help you minimize some problems (such as sleep apnea and chronic heart disease) and have more energy and a greater sense of well-being in general. However, there are many diet programs available for sale that is really complex or very expensive. Therefore, creating a plan to lose your weight will be much more beneficial, since it will be something that you can maintain in the long term. Adapt this program to your lifestyle, taking into account the costs that you can face, the aspects that you like or dislike of the diets and the frequency of physical exercise. Keep these aspects in mind when creating planning to lose weight more.

Create a plan to lose weight

Ask for an appointment with your doctor. Talk to your doctor to find out exactly what your ideal weight is and how many kilos you should lose. Also, the professional will evaluate any medication you are taking or any illness you may have to determine if it is safe for you to start a weight loss plan.

Your doctor will also help you determine if your physical ability allows you to perform vigorous routines or exercises.

It will also give you basic tips when counting the calories and decide what is best for you.

Set realistic goals whenever you start a program to lose weight (bought or own), it is important that you set realistic goals. This will help you determine the type of diet, duration and physical activity (in case you need to include it) that you have to perform. In general, people who set goals that are too big are often discouraged or lose motivation, so they end up giving up. Put the plan on the calendar to motivate you.

Usually, it is not recommended to lose more than 0.5 to 1 kilo (1 to 2 pounds) per week. That is the average considered safe, realistic and sustainable to lose weight.

Diets that promise faster and greater weight loss are usually not safe or sustainable over time. Therefore, focus on smaller and achievable goals.

If you have to lose many kilos, establish several objectives. You can have a long-term goal and other small prior goals. For example, the long-term goal may be to lose 15 kilos (30 pounds) in 6 months. The short-term objectives can be to lose 2.5 kilos (5 pounds) in two weeks, 5 kilos (10 pounds) in four or five weeks, etc.

Buy or make your calendar to keep track of the objectives. Circle the start day and end day of the program. In this way, you will establish a specific deadline to reach your goals, which will mark the way forward.

You can also indicate the days you want to exercise. Make sure to mark them on the calendar.

Place the calendar in a visible place so you can always see it and not forget what you should do. If it indicates that you have to do a cardiovascular activity, do it.

Create a reward system. Setting interesting rewards will keep you motivated throughout the program. Make sure they are specific and special things you reserve only for when you reach a goal.

Set smaller rewards to reward you for reaching smaller and intermediate goals. When you achieve the greatest and long-term goals, be sure to reward yourself with a more rewarding reward.

Generally, it is not recommended that the rewards be related to food (such as dining out at a restaurant or ordering a dessert). Choose rewards not related to food, such as doing a manicure, buying clothes or a pair of new shoes, enjoying a good massage, a game of golf on your favorite court or a new book.

Plan changes in lifestyle. Whenever you try to lose weight, it is advisable to abstain from fad diets. Instead, adopt a healthier lifestyle for life.

It has been shown that it is easier to keep small changes in diet and lifestyle for a longer period. You do not want to implement big changes when losing weight since it will be unlikely that you can keep them long term.

Create a plan to lose weight

Set the daily calorie limit. Regardless of the plan to lose weight you want to start, it will be inevitable that you eliminate some calories to achieve your goals. Determine the total amount of calories you should consume per day to lose 0.5 to 1 kilo (1 to 2 pounds) per week.

Generally, you will have to eliminate or burn more calories or plan a combination to eliminate and burn between 500 and 1000 calories a day to lose 0.5 to 1 kilo (1 to 2 pounds).

To begin, calculate the number of calories you consume on a typical day that you are not on a diet. You can use an application to keep a record of meals or a calculator on the Internet to know the daily amount of calories you consume. Once you have this result, subtract between 500 and 700 calories to know approximately how many calories you should consume to lose weight.

On the internet, you can also find calculators or applications to determine the number of calories you should consume to lose weight according to your age, gender, current weight and activity level.

Measure the portions. To maintain a low-calorie diet, it is important that you consider the appropriate size of meals and snacks. If you serve or consume large portions, it will be difficult for you to lose weight.

Buy a kitchen scale or a set of measuring cups, so you do not overdo the quantities. A measure of each meal and snack to make sure you respect the stipulated limits.

Buy containers, bowls, plates and cups of a certain size to make things easier. For example, you can store your lunch in a container that holds a cup of food.

There is an appropriate size for most meals. Generally, you should consume between 85 and 110 grams (3 to 4 ounces) of protein, 1/2 cup of cut fruit or a small serving of fruit, 1 or 2 cups of green leafy vegetables and 30 grams or 1/2 cup of grains.

Plan a diet with high or moderate protein content. Depending on your choice, you will have to decide if you want to make a diet with high or moderate protein content. This is the key to developing a meal plan that you can respect without going hungry.

Some studies have shown that high-protein diets help you lose weight a little faster and keep it off long-term.

In any plan to lose weight, the ideal is to consume a portion of lean protein at each meal and snack. If you decide to eat a diet rich in protein, you may have to consume more than one serving per meal.

If you have been very hungry on previous diets, consider the idea of making a protein-rich diet plan. It has been shown that ingesting a greater amount of proteins provides a greater feeling of satiety throughout the day.

Try a diet with low or moderate carbohydrate content. Generally, meal plans are divided into two groups: low-carbohydrate diets or moderate-carbohydrate diets. Both have advantages; choose the option that best suits your lifestyle.

It has been shown that low carbohydrate diets help you lose weight faster compared to diets with moderate content in this nutrient. However, both diets have shown similar overall results when it comes to losing weight.

Low-carbohydrate diets are more restrictive. If this is easy for you and you do not miss carbohydrates, then this may be the right diet for you.

Some people feel great anxiety about consuming carbohydrates or feel that they have better results when they incorporate a moderate amount of carbohydrates every day. Again, choose the option that best suits your needs and lifestyle.

In case you decide to limit carbohydrate consumption, restrict the choices of the group of grains first (bread, white rice, pasta, cookies, etc.). Most of the nutrients in this food group can be obtained through other foods. If you want to eat a low carb diet, limit the consumption of vegetables with starch (legumes, potatoes, winter squash and peas).

Incorporate fruits and vegetables in your meals. There are many styles of diet available. However, the majority consists of consuming several servings of fruits and vegetables per day.

Both fruits, including vegetables, are low-calorie and very nutritious foods. They contain a wide variety of vitamins, minerals, antioxidants and fibers.

Consume one or two servings of fruits per day at most. If you want to eat a low carb diet, you should eat less.

Consume approximately five servings of vegetables per day. Again, if you want to eat a low-carbohydrate diet, choose non-starchy vegetables instead of carbohydrate-rich vegetables (such as potatoes, peas, or carrots).

Drink moisturizing liquids every day. A very important aspect when preparing a plan to lose weight is to take into account the adequate consumption of water and other moisturizing liquids. This will improve your general health status and allow you to control your appetite.

To begin with, a good rule of thumb is to drink eight glasses of water per day. Nevertheless, you may require up to 13 glasses a day. The exact amount will depend on your gender, weight and level of physical activity.

Buy a bottle of water to keep track of the number of fluids you drink per day.

Incorporate exercise into your daily routine. To lose weight, it is important to incorporate physical activity into your daily routine. Have in mind that modifying your diet and starting a physical activity at the same time can be a bit overwhelming. If possible, try to modify one thing at a time.

Some studies have revealed that regular physical activity promotes weight loss and long-term maintenance.

It is recommended to incorporate 150 minutes of aerobic activity per week and two sessions of 20 minutes of strength training per week.

If you have not done physical activity for a long time, start slowly. Gradually increase the amount of time recommended during the first weeks or months.

Consider the option of starting a commercial or supervised diet plan. If you do not want to create your meal plan, you can start a commercial or supervised diet. You can also base your plan on any of the following diets:

Diet heavy in proteins and low in carbohydrates. Some commercial programs are based on a pattern of few carbohydrates and many proteins. Generally, this type of diet provides quick results, but it is difficult to maintain over time due to its restrictive nature.

Low-fat diet this particular eating pattern consists of limiting the fat content of the diet. Specifically, most low-fat diets limit the consumption of Trans and saturated fats but allow the intake of healthy fats for the heart.

Mediterranean diet. This type of eating pattern consists of consuming fruits, vegetables, whole grains, fish and small amounts of animal protein (beef or poultry). It has been proven to be a healthy option for those who suffer from heart problems and can help prevent heart disease.

Find out more about medical programs for weight. Health professionals and dietitians provide these feeding plans. Generally, these diets consist of following restrictive planning or consuming low-calorie, high-protein replacements for a short period. Also, you may have to accompany this treatment with prescription medication or supplements or injections of vitamins to help suppress appetite and increase energy.

Maintain long-term weight

Some studies have shown that people who keep track of their meals tend to respect the diet more and maintain their long-term achievements. Regardless of your diet, keep track of your meals to increase your chances of success.

You can also make track of your progress. Record your weight and total weight loss weekly.

You can also write down what are the things that work and which do not. When re-evaluating the plan, reread the notes and make the necessary changes.

Re-evaluate the plan every month. Whether you decide to make a commercial diet or create a personal plan, it is important to reassess progress regularly. This will enable you to decide if the plan is working for you.

Evaluate weight loss, Weigh yourself weekly and add how many kilos you have lost throughout the month. If the results are positive, you can continue with the same plan. If you have not lost much weight, reread your food diary and the number of calories to make the necessary changes.

Evaluate how easy it has been to follow the plan. Have your meals given you physical satisfaction? Do you feel hungry throughout the day? Do you have a lot of anxiety and desire to eat? Make changes, if necessary.

Create a support group. Look for a support group while trying to lose weight and maintain it in the long term, leading a healthy lifestyle. A support group will allow you to maintain long-term weight loss.

Many studies have shown that people who have a support group or with the company of their friends, family or even other dieters have been more successful and have managed to maintain weight in the long term.

Talk to your friends, family, neighbor and co-workers about your new diet. Ask them if they would love to join.

You can also find support groups on the internet. If you prefer, look for a group that has personal encounters.

Tips

Some people do not like the taste of water. If this is your case, add some slices of lime or lemon to the water to give it a little flavor. In this way, you will also get the benefits of vitamin C.

If you find it hard to count calories, place the portions you would normally eat on your plate. Then, use a knife and fork to cut the food in half (each main course, each garnish and even drinks, except water or milk). Place the other half on a plate, cover it with aluminum foil and store it in the refrigerator.

When you go to the supermarket, check each product that you place in the shopping cart and ask yourself: "Will this help me lose weight?" If the answer is no, put it back on the shelf.

If you are too busy to train, incorporate exercises in your commitments and activities. If you need to go to the supermarket, try to walk to the nearest store and buy only what you need. If you have to drive to attend a meeting in the city, arrive a little earlier than agreed. Park a few blocks away and climb the stairs instead of taking the elevator.

Weigh yourself every day. This will allow you to stay on course and be updated regarding your progress. However, remember that the weight can vary between 1 and 2 kilos per day. Therefore, do not be surprised if the numbers oscillate.

Chapter 9- Emotions and eating, and how can we change to feel better about ourselves

Change is hard. Whenever you make any type of change to your diet, especially if your goal is the development of lifelong, healthy habits, you will find that along the way you will need some encouragement, advice, and strategy to help you get started, and also get through the rough spots that are inevitable. From navigating the grocery store to dealing with social circumstances, here are a few tips that will help you attain DASH Diet success.

- You can't start on a new path without an awareness of where you have been, or you run the risk of going backwards. The best way to begin the DASH Diet, or really any eating plan, is take an honest look at your current eating habits. Use a food journal and record everything you eat and drink for several days. Take it a step further and analyze vital nutritional content, including sodium intake. This will give you a clean look at how you need to modify your current way of eating to be in line with DASH guidelines.

- Don't do everything at once. Major changes take time, and if you keep this in mind, you are more likely to be successful with your new dietary lifestyle. Begin by making one or two small changes at a time, and keep with them until they begin to feel natural, before making more changes. For example, switch to lower fat dairy this week and work on adding more produce next week. Gradually increase servings of those fresh fruits and vegetables by adding on serving to one meal a day, for example. Not only will making these changes gradually be good for your mental commitment, it will help your body adjust to the increase in fiber and the slight detoxification you get from eliminating processed foods and extra sodium.

- Familiarize yourself with portion sizes. So, you know that one serving of meat is three to four ounces and that you need to consume four to five servings of vegetables, but do you really understand what that looks like, and how consuming those amounts of foods will make you feel in terms of satiety? Understanding what portion sizes look and feel like will go a long way in helping you follow DASH Diet guidelines.

- If you do not already, start incorporating some form of physical activity. You do not have to go full force, high endurance workout. An evening walk is just fine. As you increase the amount of fiber in your diet, you are likely to experience some bloating and gas. A little movement will go a long way in helping ease those symptoms, not to mention that if weight loss is your goal, physical activity will boost your results.

- Don't be afraid to ask questions when you are dining out or enjoying dinners and parties at a friend's house. Ask how foods are prepared and what ingredients they contain. If you plan on doing DASH for life, there will likely be an occasion here or there where you just let the plan slide, however if you live a lifestyle that has you frequently involved in entertaining or eating out, you need to step up and ask these questions to eliminate the risk of sabotaging your diet. If you are not comfortable letting your host know of your dietary restrictions, then offer to bring a dish or two to pass around. This will ensure that you also have something to enjoy and does not inconvenience anyone.

- Beware of condiments and sauces as these are often heavy in salt, sugar, and fats. Even the most unassuming ones — such as ketchup — can add milligrams of salt and unwanted sugar to your diet. Ask for foods to be prepared without extra sauces or have them served on the side so that you are in charge of how much you consume.

- Accept that you are human. DASH can be a lifelong approach to healthy eating and wellness protection as long as you are realistic about your expectations. There is room for moderation in this dietary plan; the main focus should not be on sacrifice, but on making healthy choices **most** of the time. Allow yourself an occasional treat, your mind and body will both thank you for it.

- If your finances allow, invest in some good quality cookware and kitchen utensils. The right cookware will make preparing DASH meals easier, less messy, and they will taste better also. Think about non-stick cookware that eliminates the need for excess cooking oils, vegetable steamers, and rice cookers, to make preparation effortless, and good quality spice mills for all of the flavorful and exotic new spices you will be experimenting with as you change your priorities from salty to flavorful.

- Always read labels. Always. Pay particular attention to saturated fat, sodium, and fiber content. When something appears to be high in sodium or fats, weigh what you will be giving up against what you gain from one portion of that food and ask yourself if it is worth it. In some cases, you may feel that it is. In others, the idea of giving up several servings of other foods for just one of this food will be enough to persuade you to put it down and move on to something else.

- Don't be afraid to modify your recipes. DASH isn't about putting your favorites away forever; it is about modifying them so that you can still enjoy them whenever you want without worrying that you are damaging your health. Make lower fat substitutions, reduce the amount of meat while increasing the amount of grains or vegetables, and reduce the amount of sugar and salt while making ingredient choices that enhance the flavor. For instance, add sugar free applesauce to reduce the sugar content in a muffin recipe, or a nice spice blend to help you forget that you hardly used any salt in your treasured stew recipe.

- Look at new ways of preparing foods. If you love fried foods, you can try oven frying those foods using olive oil and a whole wheat breading. Consider using low sodium broth instead of heavy oils for sautéing and learn how to steam, bake and sauté your favorite foods. These preparations are not only healthier; they are easy and require little clean up.

- Never allow yourself to go hungry, because when you are hungry you are more likely to indulge in the very foods you are trying to cut out of your life. If you find that you are hungry immediately after a meal, then your portions are too small, and you should bulk up your meals a little bit. Keep plenty of fresh snacks available to help curb hunger between meals.

- Drink plenty of water. Make sure to get in at least 8-10 glasses per day.

- Never go to the grocery store hungry. Either do your grocery shopping after a meal, or keep a healthy snack (such as fruit or vegetables) in your car to nibble before you go in. If you are not hungry, you are more likely to stick with your dietary plan rather than splurging on things that provide you with no nutrition and too much salt and fat.

- Discover the art of meal planning. There are two schools of thought on meal planning. Some people love it and enjoy devoting time to it. The other school of thought centers around the idea that it is just too much work and never works out anyway. I am here to tell you that there actually is a happy medium between these two. Even if you are not a fan of meal planning, start by planning half of your meals, even if it is just breakfast or lunch. Write out a menu, and what ingredients you need. Maybe a weekly meal plan for breakfast will only include oatmeal, eggs, low fat yogurt, fresh berries, and asparagus. But you will know each day what you will be having, which helps you commit to actually giving yourself time for preparation and you will also know that you have everything you need for each of those meals. Start small and build on it. Soon, you will find that meal planning not only makes grocery shopping easier and is gentler on the wallet, but you will begin to look forward to certain meals throughout the week. This will also help you stay on track with diet. If you are unsure of where to start with meal planning, there are several apps and websites that are helpful in creating simple weekly meal plans.

- Choose fresh whenever possible. When fresh produce is an option, choose it over canned. Frozen produce is also an excellent option as there is not the same sodium content as in canned goods. Speaking of frozen foods, limit your choices to frozen vegetables and fruits while staying away from frozen prepared meals and snacks. If you are really craving those frozen jalapeno poppers, make your own by stuffing fresh peppers with low fat cheese and spices. There is a healthy alternative to just about everything; there is no need to depend on the frozen food section for your favorite snacks and meals.

- Make it from scratch. When you make your own sauces, salad dressings and soups you are ensuring that your food contains natural, fresh ingredients with a sodium and fat content that is much less than what you will find in their prepackaged counterparts.

- If you do choose canned goods, rinse off the contents whenever possible. This especially applies for canned vegetables and meats.

- Learn to shop the perimeter of the store. This is where you will find the foods that are promoted on the DASH Diet plan. Along the perimeter, or outside aisles of your grocery store, you will find fresh produce, meat, and seafood, dairy and possibly a bakery where you can purchase fresh, whole grain breads. Save the middle aisles for things such as additional grains and spices only.

- Flavor isn't just about the spice aisle. Yes, we make the point repeatedly about choosing other spices over salt. But you should also consider other foods that add incredible flavor to your dishes, like onion, garlic, fresh ginger, citrus, vinegars, and low sodium sauces.

- Have a support system. Even better, have a multi-leveled support system. Get your family and friends involved in your decision and ask someone to be your accountability partner. These are the people that you will go to in times when you have difficulty sticking to the plan. We all start out with pure intentions, but when we are honest with ourselves; we know there will be times when we need a little nudge to stay on track. This is what your support is for. Also, it is helpful to have a medical support system that includes a physician or dietician that can help you along the way as you encounter questions or require evaluation.

- Finally, reward yourself for a job well done, and forgive yourself when things don't go as planned. What are the things you dreamed about doing or accomplishing once you became healthier or lost some weight? Was it a new outfit, the confidence to finally join that group fitness class, or run a half marathon, or take that spa trip with friends that you always found a way to talk yourself out of? These are the types of things you should reward yourself with as you reach your personal goals. But also, be gentle with yourself. You are setting out on a new road, and along the way there will be bumps and you may feel shaken enough to jump off the path. You are more likely to stay true to your goals when you allow yourself to make a few mistakes. The process of changing your lifestyle is long term, and it is an ongoing learning adventure. When you have a slip up, evaluate what caused it and learn from your mistake. Forgive yourself, dust yourself off, and carry on. This is the path to success.

Conclusion

Today, the kind of lifestyle we live is altogether different from what our precursors had. With the invasion of technology into our lives, we are getting busier and our life is full of pressure and stress and some of it likewise relies upon the manner in which we eat and what we eat.

The word DASH really implies Diet Approaches to Stop Hypertension. It is advanced by the National Institute of Health, which is a United States government association. The word DASH itself is self-explanatory that the DASH diet is mainly to control hypertension. Currently, around 50 million people are influenced by hypertension in the United States and roughly one billion around the world. The relationship between blood pressure and cardiovascular infection events stays predictable. Hence, there are greater chances of events like heart attack, heart failure, heart stroke, and other kidney infections. Dieting and keeping up fitness may just lift our muscular strength, yet it can't bring down the risk of such events. If a person is experiencing hypertension, his body won't respond much to his fitness routine, so it is significant for us to deal with both muscular and scholarly organs.

One of the real highlights of the DASH diet is restricting the admission of sodium, and consumption of nuts, entire grains, fish, poultry, foods grown from the ground. DASH Diet likewise encourages bringing down the consumption of red meats, desserts, and sugar. DASH diet food is rich in potassium, magnesium, calcium, protein, and fiber. The diet means to reduce to the systolic and diastolic blood pressure in patients, in the meantime giving them a day by day caloric admission of 1699 to 3100 dietary calories. Since the DASH diet includes a high quotient of hostile to oxidant rich foods, it can avert ceaseless health issues like malignancy, heart illnesses, and stroke.

With high hope for people to lower their blood pressure by being on the DASH diet; an ever increasing number of people are following this new pattern in dieting. By being on the DASH diet; you won't just lower your blood pressure; you will likewise, extraordinarily, decrease your danger of coronary illness.

Besides, this diet has been prescribed by the American Heart Association, for the individuals who have heart inconvenience or high blood pressure and are looking for an approach to eating well diet. In the event that this is you; you are in karma since this diet can likewise assist you with losing weight and live more.

In the event that you don't have the foggiest idea what DASH implies; it is the abbreviations for Dietary Approaches to Stop Hypertension. Furthermore, this diet is known to lower the blood your blood pressure, inside 14 days of being on it.

Additionally, in the diet; you are given rules on the most proficient method to eat well and on the measure of servings of sustenance you ought to eat a multi-day. The main goal of this diet is to raise the level of the intake of minerals, for example, magnesium, calcium, and potassium.

The expanded intake of vegetables, while on this diet, is additionally significant, which thusly, will diminish the need to eat unfortunate foods. As a result of this diet; weight loss will happen, due to the reducing of calorie intake. This diet is likewise against the intake of a lot of sodium-rich and handled foods, which will raise your blood pressure, along these lines making the diet ineffectual. This is the reason such foods ought to be constrained and the focus ought to be on eating whole grain and high fiber foods.

Shockingly, the Mayo Clinic has embraced this soil, which, for the most part, bolsters a diet, loaded up with a lot of grapefruit eating and drinking. In the event that you are hoping to discover increasingly about the DASH diet; you should discover a book titled, "The DASH Diet Action Plan," by Marla Hiller. This book has everything you have to think about DASH dieting and can help you on your approach to lowering your blood pressure and losing a lot of weight.

Likewise, with all diets, this isn't intended to be a long haul arrangement. Pursue a diet carefully as plot and insofar as recommended. Don't overdo it and stop it when the diet plan closes or when you don't feel well or don't perceive any results whatsoever. Continuously counsel your specialist first.